The Texas Controversy Over the Cervical Cancer Vaccine

Abstract:

When GARDASIL, a vaccine protecting against the Human Papillomavirus (HPV), was approved by the U.S. Food and Drug Administration in June 2006, it sparked political and social debate among legislatures as well as advocacy groups. By drafting and submitting legislation for the mandatory vaccination against HPV for middle school girls in Texas on November 14th 2006, Representative Jessica Farrar (D- Houston) officially began the legislative process in the Texas House of Representatives. In response, tension and protest among political conservatives, religious advocacy groups, parental rights groups, as well as Merck — the pharmaceutical company responsible for the development and sale of the drug — ensued. Proponents championed the pro-life capabilities while opposition groups questioned the drugs alleged safety despite the findings in studies conducted by Merck. The pharmaceutical giant's modus operandi of lobbying states to implement the use of its drug raised suspicion, as well as, the disclosed and undisclosed cash disbursements to interest groups and politicians. The issuance of the Executive Order by Governor Rick Perry of Texas to pilot state monies toward the purchase and administration of GARDASIL, proved only to intensify the already volatile situation. This method bypassed the normal legislative process, raising questions about the infringement on the democratic process. Inevitably, as the quagmire between social responsibility and political ideologies unfolds, the options for reaching a consensus may prove to be limited. Yet, as competing opponents and proponents strive to make their interests heard, their demands will not cease until a compromise is reached.

Introduction

On June 8th 2006, Merck & Company Incorporated announced that the U.S. Food and Drug Administration (FDA) approved GARDASIL, the first and only vaccine to prevent cervical, vulvar, and vaginal pre-cancers caused by the Human Papillomavirus (HPV) types 6, 11, 16 and 18.[1] Given that in the United States, approximately 10,000 women are diagnosed with cervical cancer every year, and an average of 10 women die each day from the disease, Merck sees this vaccination as a positive step in improving public health.

The controversy erupted on February 2nd, 2007, when Texas Republican Governor, Rick Perry issued Executive Order RP65 (see appendix-1) mandating that beginning September 2008, girls entering the sixth grade be vaccinated against HPV. The decision was not well received by the Governor's overwhelmingly conservative base as it dealt with the taboo issue of sexual health. Since the vaccination protects against sexually transmitted infection (STI), religious conservatives argue that mandating it may promote pre-marital sexual relations among young girls. Parents' groups are concerned that the decision interferes with parental discretion. Two days after signing the executive order, and in response to the wave of opposition, Governor Perry issued this statement, "Providing the HPV vaccine doesn't promote sexual promiscuity anymore than providing the Hepatitis B vaccine promotes drug use. If the medical community developed a vaccine for lung cancer, would the same critics oppose it claiming it would encourage smoking?"[2]

Medical Aspects of HPV

Definition: *Papillomaviruses are DNA tumor viruses that are widely distributed throughout animal species; these viruses are species specific. The papillomavirus that infects humans is called human papillomavirus, or HPV.*[3]

HPV is the most common STI in the United States. In the 1990s, countless epidemiologic studies have shown a consistent association between cervical cancer and HPV. There are more than 100 different strains of HPV and strains 16 and 18 are the most common high-risk strains. Thirty out of the 100 strains of HPV can potentially lead to cervical cancer. Approximately, 70% of cervical cancer cases and 90% of genital warts cases are linked to these four strains of HPV.[4]

Over half of sexually active women and men are infected with HPV at some point in their lives. In most cases, infections with HPV are not serious. Usually infections are transient, asymptomatic and resolved without treatment. However, with some individuals, HPV infections result in abnormalities in Pap tests, genital warts or, rarely, cervical cancer. Early detection and treatment of pre-cancerous lesions can prevent the development of cervical cancer, and the Pap test is the most common tool in early detection of cervical cancer.

Approximately 15% of the population in the United States between the ages of 15 and 49 are currently infected with HPV.[5] Half of the 20 million Americans infected with HPV are sexually active adolescents and young adults between the ages of 15 to 24. A number of prospective studies conducted primarily in young women have defined the following as risk factors for HPV acquisition: (1) young age (less than 25 years), (2) increasing number of sex partners, (3) early age at first sexual intercourse (16 years or younger), and (4) male partner has (or has had) multiple sex partners.[6] The estimated new cases and deaths from cervical cancer in the United States in 2007 are 11,150 and 3,670, respectively.[7] Several risk factors have been identified that appear to be associated with HPV persistence as well as the progression of cervical cancer. Yet, the single most important factor associated with invasive cervical cancer is never or rarely being screened for the disease.

HPV: National Legislation

On October 24th, 2000, President Clinton signed into law the Breast and Cervical Cancer Prevention and Treatment Act of 2000 (Public Law 106-554). In December of 2000, Congress passed Public Law 106-554 which included provisions concerning HPV. When Public Law 106-555 was signed, it gave states the option to provide medical assistance through Medicaid to eligible women who were screened through the Centers for Disease Control and Prevention's (CDC) National Breast and Cervical Cancer Early Detection Program (NBCCEDP) and found to have breast or cervical cancer, including pre-cancerous conditions.[8]

In June 2006 the Advisory Committee in Immunization Practices' (ACIP) recommendation that girls ages 11 and 12 receive vaccinations resulted in a flurry of state legislation. The ACIP consists of 15 experts in fields associated with immunization who are selected by the Secretary of the U. S. Department of Health and Human Services to provide advice and guidance to the Secretary, the Assistant Secretary for Health, and the CDC on the most effective means to prevent vaccine-preventable diseases. Even after approval by ACIP, school vaccination requirements are decisions made mostly by state legislatures.

The National Vaccine Information Center (NVIC) adamantly disapproved of ACIP's 2006 recommendation urging the use of GARDASIL for all pre-adolescent girls. NVIC contends that Merck's clinical trials did not prove the HPV vaccine could be safely administered to young girls. Fueling this skepticism, are negative side effects such as severe headaches, temporary loss of vision, and dizziness that have been reported in the District of Columbia and 20 other states. Nonetheless, these reports failed to signal distress with the relevant authorities. According to the American Cancer Society, such types of side effects reported are not cause for alarm. "We have not been informed of an instance that would call into question the overall safety of the vaccine,"[9] said Debbie Saslow, Director of Breast and Cervical Cancer Control at the American Cancer Society. Likewise, the CDC conceded that it will not alter its approval of the vaccine despite the number of adverse events revealed through the reporting system.

Texas Takes Notice of HPV

As a result of the ACIP recommendation on HPV vaccination, numerous state legislatures began introducing legislation focusing on this emerging public health issue. On November 14, 2006 Representative Jessica Farrar (D-Houston) filed HB 215 in the House of Representatives mandating the HPV vaccine be administered to girls "at an appropriate age" as a requirement to enroll in school.[10] Identical companion legislation, SB 110, was also filed the same day in the Senate by Senator Leticia Van de Putte (D-San Antonio) who is Chair of the Veteran Affairs and Military Installations Committee and sits on the Senate Committees on Education, State Affairs, and Business and Commerce. Bill HB 215 was first read on January 30, 2007 and sent that day to the Public Health Committee. After working for almost 2 ½ months to garner support for the bill,

Representative Farrar and Governor Perry both felt that it did not have a strong likelihood of passing after being informed that the bill would not be read in committee. Three days later, on February 2nd, Governor Perry issued Executive Order RP65 which came as a surprise to Democrats and Republicans alike.

The order stipulates that the Department of Health and Human Services move with all speed to implement a vaccination program. It also requires the legislature to work on funding for the initiative. For those who may have moral or ethical objections to the vaccination, the executive order allows for the possibility to opt out of participation upon completion of the necessary paperwork.

Numerous members of the 80th Texas legislature not only opposed the order but questioned whether the Governor was overstepping the boundaries of his executive power by advocating for vaccination through a decree as opposed to abiding by the normal legislative process. According to the Texas Constitution, the lawmaking process begins in either the House or Senate where a legislator drafts a bill and sends it to the chamber floor for debate and/or amendments. The bill must receive a two-thirds majority vote in order to be passed along to the other chamber for consideration. The proposed bill undergoes deliberation, up to three committee readings, and needs a two-thirds majority vote to pass. Once a bill has been voted on and approved by both the House and Senate, it is signed by the respective leaders of both chambers and sent to the Governor's desk for the final stages of approval before becoming a law. Consequently, the Governor has 10 days from the time the bill is presented to either approve it, by signing it into law, or veto it at which time it is sent back to the chamber from which it originated. If the bill is not signed or vetoed by the Governor by the end of 10 days, it becomes law. The legislature can override the Governor's veto if the bill receives a two-thirds majority in both the House and Senate (see appendix 2).[11]

There is heavy debate regarding the weight of this executive order under Texas law, explains Janet Elliott, a writer for the Houston Chronicle and San Antonio Express. Opponents of the HPV vaccination mandate argue that Governor Perry stepped outside the bounds of his legal authority in issuing this order and as Elliot explains, "the State Attorney General put out the word that Perry exceeded his authority but is not issuing a written opinion."[12] This law is not set to take effect until September 2008 which raises questions among critics about the alleged sense of urgency associated with the matter as justification for bypassing the normal legislative process.

Two major bills have been sponsored within the Texas legislature in hopes of pre-empting the Governor's mandate. On February 5th, 2007, Senator Hegar Glenn Hager (R-Katy) filed bill SB 438 with the support of numerous other members of legislature including Senator Jane Nelson (R-Lewisville).[13] The bill seeks to prohibit the requirement of the HPV vaccination for admission to elementary and secondary school. If passed by both chambers, this bill still runs the risk of veto by Governor Perry, in which case, a two-thirds majority in both chambers would be required to override the veto before the end of the 80th legislature's regular session on May 28th. There is still debate over whether the passage of this bill would override the weight of the Governor's executive order and the issue is being analyzed by the State Attorney General and other legal experts.

On February 9th, Senator Hager, Vice-Chair of the Committee on Government Organization and member of the Nominations Committee, threatened to withhold support for Perry's nomination of Albert Hawkins as Commissioner of the Health and Human Services Commission until he explains how he intends to implement Perry's Order. "While Commissioner Hawkins is not responsible for issuing the order to mandate the use of GARDASIL in every 11 and 12 year old girl in the State of Texas, he is indeed the person who is responsible for developing and ultimately approving the plan to carry out the Governor's order" Hegar said.[14]

House Representative Jessica Farrar and Senator Leticia Van de Putte, both of whom have been working closely with Governor Perry on garnering support for HPV legislation (prior to the issuance of the Executive Order) are now concerned with ensuring accurate public information regarding the vaccine and cervical cancer. Lillian Ortiz, a legislative assistant to State Representative Farrar, explains that the main focus should now be ensuring the passage of a bill that would require medically accurate information to parents who may not be totally informed on the subject. She emphasized the importance of a bill focused on accurate education as a first step toward an eventual mandatory HPV vaccination. Representative Farrar, herself, goes on to explain, "The medically accurate part may seem like a no-brainer, but in Texas because this is something that has to be very much monitored because we've had past experiences that have resulted in misinformation being put out as official state health information."[15] She cites the Women's Right to Know brochure as one example where an educational pamphlet required for women choosing to have an abortion, misrepresented medical facts and associated abortion with a higher incidence of breast cancer. The conservative base's influence on the political agenda and occasional hegemony over information presented to the public is a powerful and influential attribute of the Texas legislature.

Governor Rick Perry

Rick Perry's life seems to parallel that of the "American Dream." Born in 1950, Perry grew up on the periphery of public life watching his father serve as a school board member and as Haskell County Commissioner. He began his political career in 1984 as a Democrat when he won a seat in the Texas House of Representatives from a rural district in West Texas.[16] After being passed up for a leadership position in 1989 he promptly switched parties and continued to serve as a representative until 1991.[17] It was then that he moved into his first statewide elected position where he served two terms as the Texas Commissioner of Agriculture. In 1998, he was elected Lieutenant Governor. He served in this capacity until then Governor George W. Bush was declared President by the U.S. Supreme Court. Rick Perry was sworn in as Governor of Texas on December 21, 2000.[18] Later elected to a full term in 2002 and another in 2006, Perry's social and fiscal policies have never been questioned to be anything but conservative.

Due to the fact that the Lieutenant Governor presides over the state Senate, controls its proceedings, and holds the power to appoint committee members and chairs, many in Texas consider it more powerful than the office of the Governor.[19] In 2006, Perry won a hard fought election for his second full term in which he only won with a plurality of 39% of the vote.[20] Political consultant, Bill Miller sees the Governor's HPV Executive Order as, "an example of the Governor going his own way without political consequences. He has immunity at the ballot box."[21] Other political observers have taken that observation a step further and speculate that Perry could be using the executive order, "to raise his national profile as a potential vice presidential candidate."[22] Regardless, it is widely believed that his wide use of executive orders and record-setting use of vetoes are both attempts at strengthening the office of the Governor.[23]

Aside from strengthening his office it remains unclear why Governor Perry chose to issue an executive order on this issue. Clearly he has alienated his socially conservative base. Surprisingly, he has found much more support on the other side of the aisle as many Democrats feel that from a policy standpoint, the order is smart public health policy. To many the issue remains, however, whether or not the Governor overstepped his bounds by sidestepping the democratic process and mandating that tax monies be spent on a program without taxpayer input. Senator Jane Nelson and Representative Jim Keffer (R- Eastland), himself a supporter of the vaccine and Chair of the House Ways and Means Committee, asked Attorney General Greg Abbott to issue an opinion on the weight of the executive order. According to a joint statement issued March 12, 2007:

> "The Attorney General met with both of us, and he answered questions we had regarding the executive order. It appears that RP 65 is, in effect, an advisory order and does not carry the weight of law. The Health and Human Services Commissioner is not required to follow the order. Additionally, a governor cannot, through executive order, direct an agency to do something it does not already have the authority to do."[24]
> - Senator Jane Nelson, R-Lewisville, & Representative Jim Keffer, R-Eastland

One thing that does appear certain is the impact Perry's personal life has played in his decision to issue the executive order. He has acknowledged that cancer has affected many in his family and that he will do everything he can to fight the disease. He has even proposed the sale of the Texas Lottery (another widely unpopular proposal) to help fund cancer initiatives. Perry's wife, Anita, a nurse and the daughter of a doctor, has been a strong proponent of the order as well and has attended Women in Government functions as a keynote speaker on the ills of cervical cancer.

Prior to the issuance of the executive order, Governor Perry had been working closely with Representative Jessica Farrar on legislation HB 215 that would have required the vaccination for all girls "at an appropriate age."[25] According to Representative Farrar, if the Senate passes any bill prohibiting the HPV vaccine, it will be the only vaccine prohibited from ever appearing on the list of vaccines required to enroll in school unless a future legislature decided to mandate it. Texas law leaves the required vaccine decision to the Texas Health and Human Services Commission.

Merck

Established in 1891, Merck & Co. has become a global research-driven pharmaceutical company committed to the discovery, development, marketing and manufacturing of medicines and vaccines. In 1995, Merck and CSL Limited entered into a licensing agreement and begun collaborative efforts in developing the technology used to produce GARDASIL. GARDASIL, approved by the FDA in 2006, is Merck's third-newest vaccine on the market. Merck has allocated millions of dollars to accelerate the availability of GARDASIL in the developing and developed worlds.

GARDASIL went under evaluation in four placebo-controlled, double-blind, randomized clinical studies. The studies reviewed and documented the results from 20,541 women ages 16 to 26 exposed to the drug. Study participants were then followed for up to five years. These studies suggest that exposure to GARDASIL, for women who are previously infected with one or more HPV strains prior to vaccination, protected them from the virus caused by the remaining strains but may not alter the course of an infection already present. Even though the initial development of GARDASIL was tested on older women, previous vaccination strategies have shown that the best time to administer any vaccine is before exposure to the infection. Previous studies lead to the observation that perhaps adolescents are an important group to vaccinate against HPV; since, one in four people ages 15-24 are infected with HPV.

Merck studied the anti-HPV 6,-11, -16 and -18 immune responses for GARDASIL in 10 to 15 year-old girls and compared the findings to those of the 16 to 23 year-old adolescent and young adult women. Merck found that there was no significant difference in the immune responses of participants who received GARDASIL. These analyses were fundamental to the FDA approval for the use of GARDASIL by girls ages 9 to 15.

Since the FDA's approval of GARDASIL and the ACIP's recommendation, Merck has devoted time and money to efforts, across the country, associated with legislation that would mandate the vaccination of young girls against HPV. It doubled its lobbying budget in Texas (Rick Perry received $6000 from Merck's Political Action Committee during his re-election campaign.[26] and created a conduit for money through the Women in Government — an advocacy group made up of female state legislators around the country. Women in Government is a bi-partisan, non-profit, educational association founded in 1988 for elected women in state government. The group sees itself as an organization that supports a neutral platform, brings policymakers together to share information and looks for solutions to pertinent issues before federal, state and local governments.

In the years following its founding, two additional components were added to Women in Government's mission. The Legislative Business Roundtable and the International Leadership Exchange were added to promote the public-private partnerships between women state policymakers and leaders in the business community. The goal of the Roundtable and Exchange was to address issues of mutual concern and promote collective problem solving. The Exchange aimed to unite women state legislators and business leaders with international government officials, women business leaders and women in various levels of government. Its intention was to create an ongoing dialogue and highlight areas of mutual concern while understanding the fundamental differences between legislators in different countries.

As a result of its partnership with Merck, Women in Government has made cervical cancer elimination one of its top priorities. Despite the implied connection between Women in Government and Merck, Susan Crosby, President of the group, said that the organization receives "unrestricted" grants from Merck and that Women in Government determines the content of its educational efforts. Possibly attributed to aggressive lobbying tactics or marketing, Merck recorded sales of GARDASIL totaling $235 million at the end of 2006. However, the Women in Government President insists that Merck has its "own marketing team," adding that "We don't go hand-in-hand with a lobbyist to talk to a legislator." [27]

Merck spokeswoman Janet Skidmore would not say how much the company is spending on lobbyists or how much it has donated to Women in Government. Crosby also declined to specify how much the drug company has given but Skidmore did say that "We (Merck) disclosed the fact that we provide funding to this organization. We're not in any way trying to obscure that." [28]

The New Jersey-based drug company could generate billions in sales if GARDASIL, at $360 for the three-shot regimen, were made mandatory across the country. The executive mandate in Texas that would require each female entering sixth grade to receive the recommended three-dose regimen is an example of GARDSASIL's profit potential. Most insurance companies now cover the vaccine, and in the case of Texas, Governor Perry has directed the state health authorities to facilitate the free availability of the drug to girls 9 to 18 who are uninsured or whose insurance does not cover vaccines. Despite solutions to resolve the cost issues associated with the vaccine, many see the relationship between Merck and Women in Government as too cozy. Although Merck's methods of lobbying through groups, like Women in Government, and meeting directly with legislators are common in state government it still raises concerns when pharmaceutical companies' agendas take priority over parental rights.

On February 20th, Merck publicly announced that it would curb its nationwide lobbying efforts to make GARDASIL mandatory for young girls' entry into 6th grade across the country. "We do not want any misperception about Merck's role to distract from the ultimate goal of fighting cervical cancer, so Merck has re-evaluated its approach at the state level and we will not lobby for school requirements for GARDASIL," explained Mary Elizabeth Blake who serves as Senior Director of Public Affairs for Merck's vaccine division.[29]

Opposition Gains Momentum

Parental Rights Groups were among the most vocally opposed to Governor Perry's decision to mandate the vaccination against HPV for all 11 year old girls. These groups, including Focus on the Family and the Pro Family Law Center, were in agreement that such a mandate infringed upon parental rights to choose how much of sexual heath issues they wanted to expose their children to. Many groups are urging the Governor to reverse his decision and are likely to support any legislation that is against requiring vaccination as a precondition for middle school admission. The Pro-Family Law Center believes that the Governor's mandate "disturbs a natural incentive for teenage students to abstain from sexual intercourse to avoid the contraction of certain sexually transmitted infections."[30] This group also cited concern about the government overstepping its boundaries by interfering with parental rights as it regards the appropriate time to raise the issue of sex.

Among those groups firmly opposed to Governor Perry's Executive Order are conservative Christian and Pro-life groups. The most notable among them is an organization called Children of God for Life headed by Debbie Vinnedge, the organization's Executive Director. Debbie argues that although the decision has an opt out clause, allowing parents to forgo the vaccination for religious purposes, the children and their parents will be singled out in school and viewed as "those people". This conservatively religious base has found itself in opposition to a Governor who espouses the same anti-abortion and anti stem-cell research stance upon which the group is founded. Wendy Wright, President of Concerned Women for America, another religious right group, says that "the Governor's order forces little girls to be shot with a sex vaccine," and claims that such a decision is "an outrageous assault on girls and their parents."[31]

Another strong critic of the Governor's Executive Order has been the Texas Eagle Forum, headed by Cathie Adams. The Texas Eagle Forum is a conservative pro-family rights group dedicated to having a participatory role in government decisions and public policy to ensure the preservation of conservative values and morals. In the past, the group has been hugely successful in lobbying Congress and affecting the direction of the policy debate. The organization's website provides a venue and detailed instructions on how to effectively lobby elected officials by writing letters and even by reaching out to media sources to voice discontent with proposed policies that go against the group's moral fabric. Adams contends that the Governor's action has robbed the State legislature of its congressional authority and is infringing on parental rights as well. When contacted by the Governor's office and asked for her backing, she expressed her staunch opposition to the mandate and her desire to see to it that it is defeated. Adams cited other reasons for her opposition including that too little is known about the side effects of the vaccination and that it may provide girls with a green light to be prematurely sexually active knowing that they are protected against HPV infection.[32] The Governor has tried to frame the issue of mandatory HPV vaccination as one of being 'pro-life' in that it saves women from cervical cancer, in hopes of appealing to his conservative base and gaining their support moving forward.

Just three days after Governor Perry signed the executive order, Senator Jane Nelson urged for its repeal. Nelson expressed her dismay at the Governor's decision to issue this executive order instead of allowing for the Legislature to come to a decision jointly. She fully advocated for time to discuss drawbacks, costs and potential benefits associated with vaccinating girls. It is not surprising that the order was met with criticism. Conservative organizations and Republican lawmakers were suspicious of the Governor's relationship, direct or indirect, with Merck & Co. Perry's former Chief of Staff, Mike Toomey, is now a lobbyist for Merck. Despite the

Governor's indirect connection, aides to the governor dismissed suspicions as absurd. Perry stands by his decision because he is confident that the vaccine will protect the health of women, and he rejects suggestions that mandating the vaccine would encourage teenage girls to have sex.

Lieutenant Governor David Dewhurst, a Republican who presides over the Texas Senate, also suggested that Perry acted with haste in not consulting with lawmakers. Perry and his aides pointed out that the order allows parents to let their children opt out of the vaccine for religious or moral reasons. Dewhurst expressed his preference for an arrangement that would allow parents to opt into the program instead. While some people may disagree about how the requirement came about, many in the medical field support the requirement and believe that, with education on the issue, more people will see the three-shot vaccine's benefits.

Senator Jane Nelson

A former public school teacher who was elected to the Texas Senate in 1992, Senator Jane Nelson has, over the years, become the second highest ranking Republican in the Texas Senate. Prior to being elected to the Texas Senate Nelson served two terms on the State Board of Education. She now serves as Chairman of the Health and Human Services Committee in the Senate. Senator Nelson has devoted much of her time to health care issues, education and business. Driven by strong conservative ideals she has sponsored such bills as "Celebrate Freedom Week" in Texas' schools and has been recognized by the state business community for her efforts to reduce the size of state government, reduce healthcare costs and tie tourism in with the state's economic development plan.

Nelson has been an extremely vocal opponent of Governor Perry's Executive Order RP65, "Executive orders should be used in extreme circumstances, during times of emergency and when the Legislature is not in session. We need to be afforded the opportunity to carefully study how this would affect our budget, parental rights, and most importantly, the health of our daughters."[33] She is co-author of SB 438 (a bill written by Senator Hager) which aims to prohibit the inoculation against HPV as a condition for admission to public schools in Texas.

To some, her intractable stance on the vaccine stands in contrast to her support for fighting cancer. In early March, Senators Nelson and Keffer announced the establishment of the Texas Cancer Research Initiative. The initiative will provide up to $300 million per year in the form of research grants and loans with the goal of reducing the occurrence of cancer in Texas. "Knowing that last week Senator Nelson and Representative Keffer stood up with Gov. Perry at a news conference about finding a cure for cancer, we hope they and other legislators will join him in making sure the first vaccine ever created that prevents a cancer will get the widest distribution possible to protect young women from this deadly virus" said Robert Black, Governor Perry's spokesman.[34]

What Next?

Those opposed to the HPV vaccine have scored major victories in recent months. These include a Health Committee 6-3 majority vote (5 Republicans and 1 Democrat) to reverse Executive Order RP65, and HB 1098 (companion legislation to Senator Hegar's bill SB 438 to prohibit a mandatory HPV vaccine) which now has 90 co-authors out of 150 House members.[35] The opponents also appear to be winning in the court of public opinion as well. Most of those who have not signed on as co-authors of HB 1098 are representatives from the Mexico border area and East Texas where the prevalence of cervical cancer is among the highest in the nation.[36] Even those who support Perry's goal of requiring the vaccine for school enrollment are beginning to suggest that he rescind it. "He created a firestorm that has taken the place of public policy. Now this decision is being made on emotion," said Rep. Garnet Coleman, a Democrat from Houston and one of the remaining House members who do not support efforts to prohibit the HPV vaccine.[37] Research shows that once parents are educated properly on HPV and the vaccine, they tend to favor vaccination. Thus, along with the fact that 81 Republicans and 69 Democrats comprise the Texas House,[38] there appears to be some hope in eventually getting the HPV vaccine included in the list of vaccine requirements for school enrollment.[39] It will not be easy and it will not be swift.

Strategic Question:

It is Friday, April 13, 2007 and you, a well-respected political consultant in Texas, have just hung up the phone with Governor Perry who is in need of your strategic expertise. Considering the various proponents and opponents of the mandate your strategy must efficiently address the various political and medical concerns associated with requiring the HPV vaccine for young girls in Texas. Knowing the facts associated with this political controversy as well as the health concerns associated with HPV, devise a strategic plan for the passage of future legislation that would redirect the current debate towards one that supports Governor Perry's initial rationale for signing the Executive Order while emphasizing the medical and educational components that support mandating HPV vaccination for school enrollment.

Appendix 1

Executive Order RP65 - February 2, 2007

Relating to the immunization of young women from the cancer-causing Human Papillomavirus.

BY THE
GOVERNOR OF THE STATE OF TEXAS
Executive Department
Austin, Texas
February 2, 2007

WHEREAS, immunization from vaccine-preventable diseases such as Human Papillomavirus (HPV) protects individuals who receive the vaccine; and

WHEREAS, HPV is the most common sexually transmitted infection-causing cancer in females in the United States; and

WHEREAS, the United States Food and Drug Administration estimates there are 9,710 new cases of cervical cancer, many of which are caused by HPV, and 3,700 deaths from cervical cancer each year in the United States; and

WHEREAS, the Texas Cancer Registry estimates there were 1,169 new cases and 391 deaths from cervical cancer in Texas in 2006; and

WHEREAS, research has shown that the HPV vaccine is highly effective in preventing the infections that are the cause of many of the cervical cancers; and

WHEREAS, HPV vaccine is only effective if administered before infection occurs; and

WHEREAS, the newly approved HPV vaccine is a great advance in the protection of women's health; and

WHEREAS, the Advisory Committee on Immunization Practices and Centers for Disease Control and Prevention recommend the HPV vaccine for females who are nine years through 26 years of age;

NOW THEREFORE, I, RICK PERRY, Governor of Texas, by virtue of the power and authority vested in me by the Constitution and laws of the State of Texas as the Chief Executive Officer, do hereby order the following:

Vaccine. The Department of State Health Services shall make the HPV vaccine available through the Texas Vaccines for Children program for eligible young females up to age 18, and the Health and Human Services Commission shall make the vaccine available to Medicaid-eligible young females from age 19 to 21.

Rules. The Health and Human Services Executive Commissioner shall adopt rules that mandate the age appropriate vaccination of all female children for HPV prior to admission to the sixth grade.

Availability. The Department of State Health Services and the Health and Human Services Commission will move expeditiously to make the vaccine available as soon as possible.

Public Information. The Department of State Health Services will implement a public awareness campaign to educate the public of the importance of vaccination, the availability of the vaccine, and the subsequent requirements under the rules that will be adopted.

Parents' Rights. The Department of State Health Services will, in order to protect the right of parents to be the final authority on their children's health care, modify the current process in order to allow parents to submit a request for a conscientious objection affidavit form via the Internet while maintaining privacy safeguards under current law.

This executive order supersedes all previous orders on this matter that are in conflict or inconsistent with its terms and this order shall remain in effect and in full force until modified, amended, rescinded, or superseded by me or by a succeeding governor.

Given under my hand this the 2nd day of February, 2007.

RICK PERRY(Signature)
Governor

Attested by:
ROGER WILLIAMS(Signature)
Secretary of State

Appendix 2 **Diagram of Legislative Process**

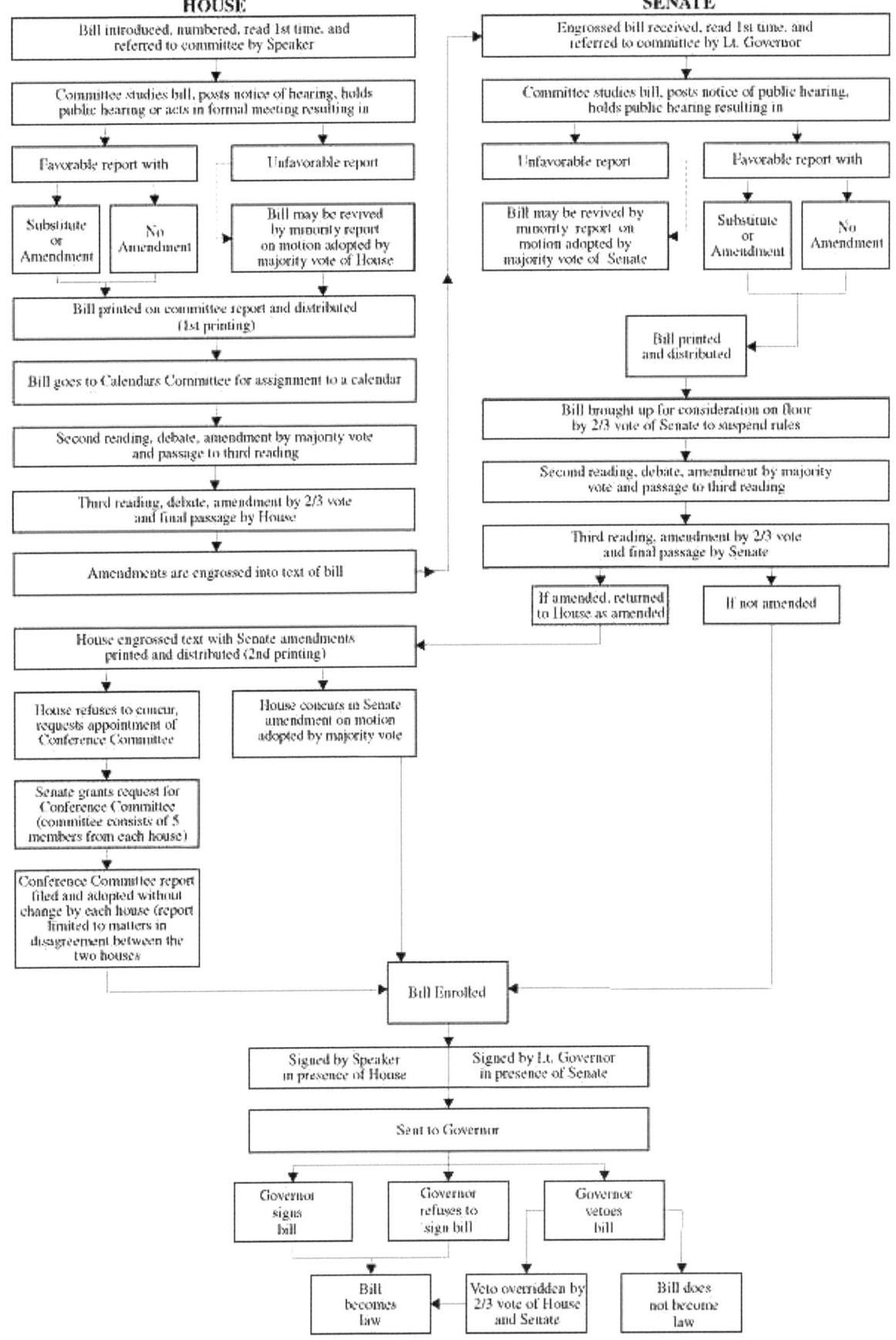

HOUSE

Bill introduced, numbered, read 1st time, and referred to committee by Speaker

Committee studies bill, posts notice of hearing, holds public hearing or acts in formal meeting resulting in

Favorable report with

Unfavorable report

Substitute or Amendment

No Amendment

Bill may be revived by minority report on motion adopted by majority vote of House

Bill printed on committee report and distributed (1st printing)

Bill goes to Calendars Committee for assignment to a calendar

Second reading, debate, amendment by majority vote and passage to third reading

Third reading, debate, amendment by 2/3 vote and final passage by House

Amendments are engrossed into text of bill

House engrossed text with Senate amendments printed and distributed (2nd printing)

House refuses to concur, requests appointment of Conference Committee

House concurs in Senate amendment on motion adopted by majority vote

Senate grants request for Conference Committee (committee consists of 5 members from each house)

Conference Committee report filed and adopted without change by each house (report limited to matters in disagreement between the two houses)

SENATE

Engrossed bill received, read 1st time, and referred to committee by Lt. Governor

Committee studies bill, posts notice of public hearing, holds public hearing resulting in

Unfavorable report

Favorable report with

Bill may be revived by minority report on motion adopted by majority vote of Senate

Substitute or Amendment

No Amendment

Bill printed and distributed

Bill brought up for consideration on floor by 2/3 vote of Senate to suspend rules

Second reading, debate, amendment by majority vote and passage to third reading

Third reading, amendment by 2/3 vote and final passage by Senate

If amended, returned to House as amended

If not amended

Bill Enrolled

Signed by Speaker in presence of House

Signed by Lt. Governor in presence of Senate

Sent to Governor

Governor signs bill

Governor refuses to sign bill

Governor vetoes bill

Bill becomes law

Veto overridden by 2/3 vote of House and Senate

Bill does not become law

Endnotes

[1] Merck's Cervical Cancer Vaccine, Gardasil®, Added to the CDC Vaccines for Children Contract November 1, 2006. Retrieved on February 20, 2007, from http://www.merck.com/newsroom/press_releases/product/2006_1101.html

[2] Perry, Rick. February 5 2007. Statement of Gov. Rick Perry on HPV Vaccine Executive Order. Retrieved on February 20, 2007, from http://www.governor.state.tx.us/divisions/press/pressreleases/PressRelease.2007-02-05.4721/view

[3] Human Papillamovirus: HPV Information for Clinicians. April 2007. Centers for Disease Control and Prevention. Retrieved on April 4, 2007 from www.cdc.gov/std/hpv/common-infection/CDC_HPV_ClinicianBro_LR.pdf

[4] Centers for Disease Control and Prevention. Epidemiology and Prevention of Vaccine-Preventable Diseases. Atkinson W, Hamborsky J, McIntyre L, Wolfe S, eds. 10th ed. Washington DC: Public Health Foundation, 2007. Retrieved on February 1, 2007 from http://www.cdc.gov/nip/publications/pink/hpv.pdf

[5] Ibid

[6] U.S. Preventive Services Task Force. January 2003. *Screening for Cervical* Cancer. Retrieved on February 1, 2007 from http://www.ahcpr.gov/clinic/uspstf/uspscerv.htm

[7] Centers for Disease Control and Prevention. Epidemiology and Prevention of Vaccine-Preventable Diseases. Atkinson W, Hamborsky J, McIntyre L, Wolfe S, eds. 10th ed. Washington DC: Public Health Foundation, 2007. Retrieved on February 1, 2007 from http://www.cdc.gov/nip/publications/pink/hpv.pdf

[8] Rollins, E., Lex, L., & Ramesh, R. June 20, 2000. S. 662-Breast and Cervical Cancer Prevention and Treatment Act of 2000. Retrieved on February 1, 2007 from http://www.cbo.gov.

[9] Lopes, Gregory. February 3, 2007. Vaccine Center Issues Warning. The Washington Times. Retrieved on February 1, 2007 from http://www.washingtontimes.com/business/20070202-100152-9747r.htm

[10] The official Website for the Texas House of Representatives. 5 Apr. 2007. The Texas House of Representatives. Retrieved on April 5 2007 from http: //www.legis.tx.us/tldocs/80R/billtext/doc/HB00215I.doc

[11] Texas Legislative Council. November 28 2006. About the Legislative Process in Texas. Retrieved February 21, 2007, from http://www.tlc.state.tx.us/gtli/legproc/process.html

[12] Janet Elliot, Personal Communication, April 6, 2007.

[13] Texas Legislature Online. History of Bill SB 438. Retrieved on March 1, 2007, from http://www.legis.state.tx.us/billlookup/History.aspx?LegSess=80R&Bill=SB 438

[14] Craven, Lisa. February 9 2007. Press Release from the Office of State Senator Glenn Hegar, D18. Retrieved on February 20, 2007, from http://www.senate.state.tx.us/75r/Senate/Members/Dist18/pr07/p020907a.htm

[15] Lillian Ortiz, Personal Communication, April 11, 2007.

[16] National Journal Website. 22 June, 2005. National Journal Group Inc. Retrieved on Feb 22. 2007. from http://nationaljournal.com/pubs/almanac/2006/people/tx/txgv.htm>.

[17] Ibid

[18] Ibid

[19] Ibid

[20] Cable News Network. Feb 27. 2007. A Time Warner Company. Retrieved on Feb 27,2007. from
http://edition.cnn.com/ELECTION/2006/pages/results/states/TX/G/00/index.html

[21] Houston Chronicle. Feb 6. 2007. Houston Chronicle Publishing Company Division, a division of Hearst Newspapers Partnership, L.P. Retrieved on Feb 10. 2007 from
http://www.chron.com/disp/story.mpl/metropolitan/4528909.html

[22] Ibid

[23] Janet Elliot, Personal Communication, April 6, 2007

[24] The official Website for the Texas Senate. March 12 2007. The Texas State Senate. Retrieved on March 15 2007. from http://www.nelson.senate.state.tx.us/pr07/p031207a.htm

[25] The official Website for the Texas House of Representatives. Apr.5 2007. The Texas House of Representatives. Retrieved on April 5 2007 from http://www.legis.tx.us/tldocs/80R/billtext/doc/HB00215I.doc

[26] Liz Austin Peterson, "Perry's office says Legislature has final say on HPV vaccine," Associated Press, February 8, 2007

[27] Crosby, Susan, President , January 30, 2007, Women in Government. Retrieved on February 5th from
http://www.news-medical.net/?id=21605

[28] Associated Press January 30, 2007. Merck lobbies states to require cervical cancer vaccine for school girls. Retrieved on February 20, 2007 from http://www.ahrp.org/cms/content/view/451/27

[29] Childs, Dan February 22, 2007. Political Intrigue in Merck's HPV Vaccine Push. ABC News Medical Unit. Retrieved on March 1, 2007, from http://abcnews.go.com/Health/story?id=2890402&page=1

[30] Unruh, Bob February 6, 2007. Family Group Compares HPV Vaccine to Condoms. World Net Daily. Retrieved on March 1, 2007, from http://www.worldnetdaily.com/news/article.asp?ARTICLE_ID=54102

[31] Associated Press February 3, 2007. Texas Governor Orders HPV Vaccine for all Girls. MSNBC. Retrieved on February 20, 2007, from http://www.msnbc.msn.com/id/16948093/wid/11915773?GT1=9033

[32] Brown, Jim February 6, 2007. Governor Perry's HPV vaccination Order angers Pro-family group. Agape Press. Retrieved on February 20, 2007, from http://www.gopusa.com/news/2007/february/0206_hpv_vaccine.shtml

[33] The official Website for the Texas Senate. Feb 20. 2007. The Texas State Senate. Retrieved on Feb 20, 2007. from http://www.nelson.senate.state.tx.us/pr07/p020507a.htm>.

[34] The Austin-American Statesman. March 13. 2007. Cox Texas Newspapers, L.P. Retrieved on March 13. 2007 from http://www.statesman.com/news/content/region/legislature/stories/03/13/13hpv.html

[35] Houston Chronicle. February 22 2007. Houston Chronicle Publishing Company Division, a division of Hearst Newspapers Partnership, L.P. Feb 22. 2007 from http://www.chron.com/disp/story.mpl/front/4571812.html>.

[36] Ibid.

[37] Ibid.

[38] Ortiz, Lillian. Personal Interview. Apr. 112007.

[39] Houston Chronicle. February 22 2007. Houston Chronicle Publishing Company Division, a division of Hearst Newspapers Partnership, L.P. Retrieved on Feb. 22 2007 from http://www.chron.com/disp/story.mpl/front/4571812.html

www.ingramcontent.com/pod-product-compliance
Lightning Source LLC
Chambersburg PA
CBHW060819290526
45792CB00005BB/1722